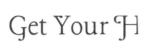

Get Your H

MW00983207

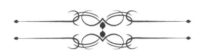

Ðaily Affirmations
for Your
Pregnancy & Childbirth

Encouraging Self-Love, Self-Care and Positive Self-Talk Ðuring Pregnancy, Childbirth and Beyond!

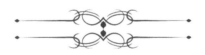

Serena A. Williams

Dedication

To my mother, who laid the foundation for my journey into motherhood. Now that I have three children of my own, I realize how much your love, guidance and support have shaped me. This book is dedicated to you, Mama, as a testament to the power of your love and the impact it has had on my life and the lives of my children. Thank you for being my role model and my rock.

I love you more than words can express.

Ðear Valued Customer,

We hope that you find our book, "Ðaily Affirmations for Your Pregnancy & Childbirth" helpful and uplifting during your pregnancy journey. Our goal is to support and encourage expectant mothers and help them feel confident and empowered throughout their pregnancy.

If you enjoy the book and find it to be beneficial, we would greatly appreciate it if you could take a moment to leave a review on Amazon. Your feedback will help others discover the book and make informed purchasing decisions. It will also contribute to the continued success and growth of our work.

Thank you for your support and for taking the time to share your thoughts with us. We truly appreciate it!

Wishing you all the best in your pregnancy journey,

Serena A. Williams
Get Your Head Right Series

Table of Contents

Introduction
Why Affirmations Matter During Pregnancy and Childbirth

Pregnancy and childbirth can be incredibly transformative experiences, both physically and emotionally. It's a time when many women experience a range of emotions, from joy and excitement to fear and anxiety. Affirmations, positive statements that are repeated often, can be a powerful tool for managing these emotions and promoting a positive mindset during this special time.

Affirmations have been used for centuries in various cultures and their effectiveness has been supported by scientific research. Studies have shown that affirmations can help reduce stress, improve mood, and increase overall well-being. For pregnant women, using affirmations can promote a sense of calm and empowerment during what can be a challenging time.

In this book, you'll find a collection of affirmations specifically designed for pregnancy and childbirth. These affirmations are intended to promote self-love, self-care, and positive self-talk during pregnancy, childbirth, and beyond. Whether you're seeking to manage anxiety, connect with your baby, or simply maintain a positive mindset throughout your pregnancy and childbirth journey, these affirmations can provide the support you need.

Take a moment to reflect on how each affirmation makes you feel and any changes or improvements you notice in your thoughts and / or feelings. By incorporating affirmations into your daily routine, you'll be able to shift your focus to the positive aspects of pregnancy and childbirth, which can help you approach these experiences with greater confidence, joy, and ease. So, let's get started on this journey and discover the power of affirmations for a positive and fulfilling pregnancy and childbirth experience.

SELF-LOVE AND SELF-CARE

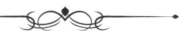

I
Have
Faith!

I am grateful for the
miracle of life
growing inside me.

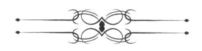

I am proud of my
growing strength and
resilience.

I am surrounded by positive energy and good vibes.

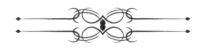

I am strong and capable of handling the physical and emotional demands of pregnancy.

I am grateful for the experience of pregnancy and the growth it brings.

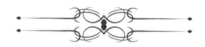

I am committed to a positive and healthy pregnancy.

I am relaxed, calm, and at peace during this pregnancy.

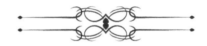

I am at peace with the changes happening in my body.

I am focusing on the positive aspects of pregnancy and motherhood.

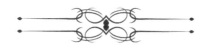

I am proud of myself for taking care of my physical and emotional health.

I am capable of advocating for myself and my baby.

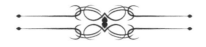

I am surrounded by positive affirmations and uplifting thoughts.

I trust my instincts
and the guidance of
my body.

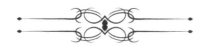

I am embracing the
changes that come
with pregnancy and
motherhood.

I am proud of the life growing inside me.

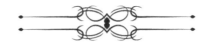

I am at peace with the unknowns of the future.

I am surrounded by
the love of my family
and friends.

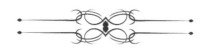

I am proud of my
growing belly and the
life it represents.

I am capable of making choices that align with my values and beliefs.

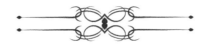

I am grateful for the opportunity to experience the miracle of life through pregnancy.

I am excited for the journey ahead and the person I will become as a mother.

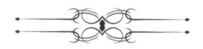

I am surrounded by the beauty of the natural world and the wonders of life.

I am proud of my strength and ability to handle whatever comes my way during pregnancy.

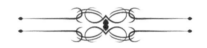

I have the resources I need during my pregnancy.

I am surrounded by the wisdom and experience of other mothers.

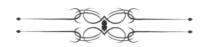

I am enjoying my pregnancy and looking forward to the journey ahead.

I will provide a safe and loving environment for my baby.

I am a beautiful pregnant woman.

I am surrounded by the warmth and comfort of my home and community.

I am grateful for the growth and transformation I am experiencing.

I am proud of my courage and determination to have a positive birth experience.

I am at peace with the unknowns of pregnancy and motherhood.

I trust my instincts to guide me during this journey.

I am capable of handling any challenges that come my way.

I trust that my pregnancy and the birth of my child will unfold as it should.

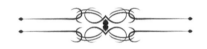

I am filled with wonder at the miracle of life growing inside of me.

I am proud of my dedication to self-care during pregnancy.

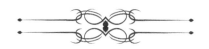

I am grateful for the journey of pregnancy and the growth it brings.

I embrace the
strength and
resilience of my body.

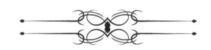

I am proud of my
courage to face any
challenges that come
my way.

I possess the strength, courage, and confidence to face this pregnancy.

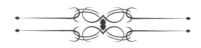

I accept all my feelings as part of who I am.

I am at peace with the ups and downs of pregnancy and the unknowns of the future.

I will give my child a happy mother.

HEALTHY PREGNANCY

I trust my body to carry and deliver my baby safely.

I am grateful for this experience and the opportunity to bring new life into the world.

I am surrounded by love and support from family and friends.

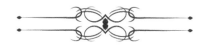

My baby is growing healthy and strong.

I am worthy of a smooth and stress-free pregnancy.

I am taking care of my body and my baby by listening to my doctor's instructions.

I am doing everything
I can to have a
healthy pregnancy
and baby.

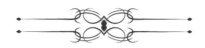

I am worthy of a
healthy and happy
pregnancy.

I am filled with love and joy as I nurture my growing baby.

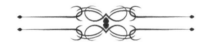

I am capable of overcoming any challenges that may arise during pregnancy.

I am proud of my body for its ability to grow and sustain a new life.

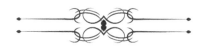

I am grateful for the love and support I receive from my community.

I am surrounded by positive energy and well wishes.

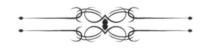

I am filled with excitement for the future and the adventures that lie ahead.

I am strong, capable,
and resilient.

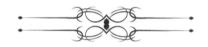

I am filled with hope
for a healthy and
happy baby.

My body is doing amazing work to bring my baby into the world.

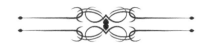

I trust my body to guide me through this pregnancy.

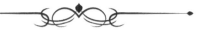

I am surrounded by positivity and encouragement.

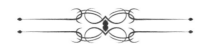

Each day, my baby and I are growing stronger and healthier.

I am taking good care of myself and my baby during this pregnancy.

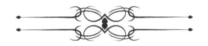

I am grateful for my body's ability to adapt.

I am committed to self-care and nurturing during my pregnancy.

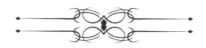

I am grateful for the growth I am experiencing during pregnancy.

I trust my body to grow and birth my baby.

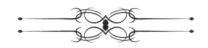

I am grateful for the journey of pregnancy and the lessons it brings.

I will adapt and overcome any obstacles during pregnancy.

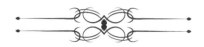

I am grateful for this beautiful journey of pregnancy.

I am creating a peaceful and loving environment for my baby to grow in.

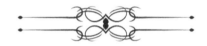

I am filled with love and happiness for my growing baby.

I am at peace with the unknowns of pregnancy and motherhood.

I deserve and will be healthy during my pregnancy.

I can handle anything
my pregnancy or
motherhood throws at
me.

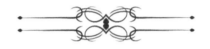

I am proud of my
strength and
resilience during this
time.

I am surrounded by love and support during this pregnancy.

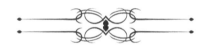

I am taking care of both myself and my growing baby.

My body is changing to give my baby what it needs.

I am proud of my body for adapting to the changes of pregnancy.

My body is designed to nourish and protect my baby.

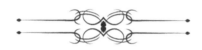

Every day my baby is growing bigger and stronger.

My baby is my greatest inspiration for living a healthy and happy life.

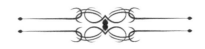

I am grateful for the journey of pregnancy and the life lessons it teaches.

CONNECTING WITH YOUR BABY

I am grateful for the bond I share with my baby.

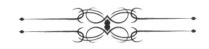

My baby and I are connected in a special way.

I love and accept my baby unconditionally.

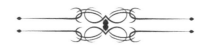

My baby is a gift.

I trust my body to nurture and care for my baby.

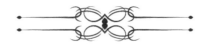

I am excited to meet my baby and hold them in my arms.

My baby is an extension of my love and compassion.

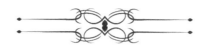

I send love and positive energy to my baby every day.

My baby hears and feels my love and connection.

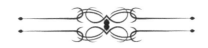

My baby's needs are important to me, and I will always prioritize their well-being.

I am attuned to my baby's needs and desires.

I am grateful for the time I get to spend bonding with my baby before birth.

My baby senses my love with each passing day.

My baby and I are in constant communication through our connection.

I feel my baby's presence with me.

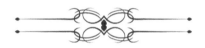

Our connection is strong and unbreakable.

I listen to my baby's needs and respond with love.

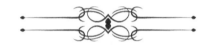

My baby and I work together for a healthy pregnancy.

My baby and I are growing and learning together.

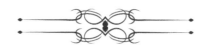

I am grateful for the opportunity to bring new life into the world.

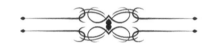

I embrace every moment of my pregnancy and cherish the bond with my baby.

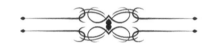

My baby and I are co-creating a beautiful life together.

I am in awe of the miracle of life growing inside of me.

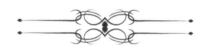

My baby is a source of joy and wonder in my life.

I am filled with love and happiness when I think of my baby.

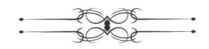

I trust that my baby is growing and developing exactly as they should.

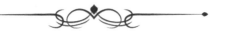

I am nurturing my baby with every breath I take.

My baby is a precious gift that I will always cherish.

I am grateful for the opportunity to bond with my baby before birth.

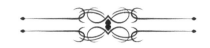

I am sending love and positive energy to my baby every day.

My baby is a source of joy in my life.

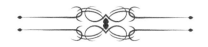

My baby and I are connected in a bond of love and protection.

I am filled with joy at the thought of holding my baby in my arms.

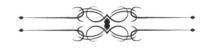

I am grateful for the bond I am forming with my baby.

My baby is safe and sound in my belly.

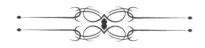

I am grateful for the opportunity to connect with my baby through touch and movement.

I am filled with love
for my baby and the
bond we share.

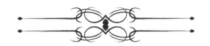

I am filled with joy at
the thought of the
first time I will see my
baby's face.

I am grateful for the time I get to spend bonding with my baby.

My connection to my baby grows stronger every day.

The bond between us
is inseparable.

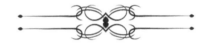

Each day I am closer
to meeting my baby.

POSITIVE BIRTH EXPERIENCE

I release any fear I have about the birth process and trust that it will unfold naturally.

I am confident in my ability to make the best decisions for my baby and myself.

I am worthy of a safe, healthy, and happy pregnancy and birth.

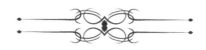

I am at peace with my choices regarding my birth plan.

I am confident in my ability to make quick and informed decisions during labor and delivery.

I am worthy of a smooth and stress-free birth.

I am patient and compassionate with myself as I move through each stage of labor.

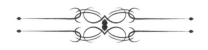

My body is strong, healthy, and capable of giving birth.

I am worthy of a healthy and happy birthing experience.

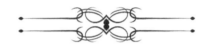

My birthing experience is unique and beautiful, just like my baby.

I am confident in my ability to give birth.

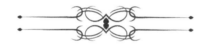

I am surrounded by a team of supportive healthcare providers.

I trust my own body to birth my baby in a safe and healthy way.

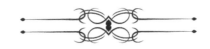

I am prepared to bring my beautiful baby into the world.

I trust that my body knows what to do during labor and delivery.

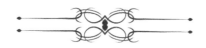

My body is relaxed and open, allowing my baby to move through with ease.

I am creating a positive and peaceful environment for my baby's birth.

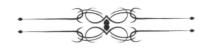

I trust the birth process and I know everything will happen as it should.

I am deeply
connected to my baby
while we work
together during labor.

My baby is coming
into this world
surrounded by love,
joy, and positivity.

I am in control of my birthing experience.

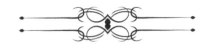

I am strong and capable of bringing new life into this world.

My body and my baby
are working together
to achieve a safe and
joyful birth.

I embrace the natural
flow of my birthing
process with ease.

My body is strong, powerful, and capable of giving birth to my baby.

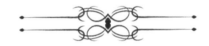

I trust my body and my baby to guide us through this journey.

Each contraction brings me closer to embracing my child.

I am safe, calm, and supported as I birth my baby.

My breath is steady,
and my mind is clear,
as I bring my baby
into the world.

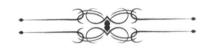

I am surrounded by
love and positivity
during my birthing
experience.

I am happy with my choices for my birth plan.

I am grateful for the opportunity to experience the miracle of birth.

I am present and I'm embracing the beauty and power of birth.

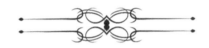

My body is designed to give birth and I trust in its natural ability to do so.

I release my fears and
I trust in the journey
of my birthing
process.

I trust my body to
know how to give
birth naturally and
beautifully.

With each breath, I
am bringing peace
and relaxation to my
body and my baby.

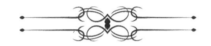

My mind is calm and
focused, and my body
is relaxed and ready
for birth.

I am surrounded by love and support as I bring my baby into the world.

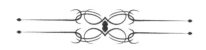

I am strong, capable, and prepared for whatever comes during my labor.

My baby is safe, healthy, and supported as they move through the birthing process.

I am grateful for the power and strength of my body, as I give birth to my child.

Each contraction brings me closer to meeting my baby.

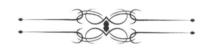

I trust my intuition and my instincts to guide me through labor and delivery.

I am open to the guidance and support of my medical team.

It's okay to change my birthing plan.

My body knows exactly what to do to give birth safely and naturally.

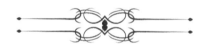

I am surrounded by love as I birth my baby.

I am relaxed and calm, allowing my body to work in harmony with my baby.

I am releasing any fear and embracing the power of birth.

I am grateful for the strength and resilience of my body throughout this journey.

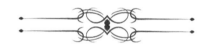

I am strong and ready for labor and delivery.

I am stronger than I think I am.

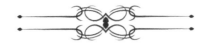

I will focus on each breath during labor.

I will be in pain but I will not be in danger.

I am stronger than my contractions could ever be.

I am bringing a
beautiful life into the
world.

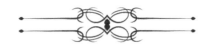

I trust in my body's
ability to give birth.

My baby is coming into this world with ease.

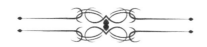

I trust that my baby will be born at the right time.

My body possess all
the strength I need to
deliver my baby.

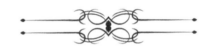

I am surrounded by
love and support from
my family and
friends.

My baby and I are a
team.

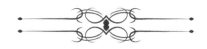

My labor will be
perfect for my baby
and I.

My life is ready for the happy addition of my little one.

I am excited to meet my baby and hold them in my arms.

ADJUSTING TO LIFE
AS A NEW PARENT

I am filled with excitement for the new challenges and adventures of motherhood.

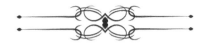

My baby is surrounded by a circle of love and protection.

I am confident in my ability to create a nurturing and stable home for my family.

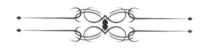

I am filled with joy at the thought of watching my baby grow and learn.

I am at peace with the uncertainty of the future and the unknowns of motherhood.

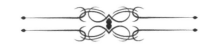

I am surrounded by loving and supportive friends and family.

I am filled with excitement for the milestones and memories to come.

I am inspired and encouraged by the women who have come before me.

I am a loving and nurturing mother.

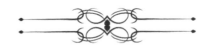

I am filled with joy at the thought of watching my baby grow and develop.

My child will prosper because I will raise them with love.

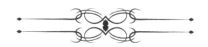

I am creating a stable and loving home for my child.

I am filled with excitement for the memories I will make with my baby.

I will provide a safe and loving environment for my baby.

I am appreciative for the experience of motherhood.

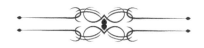

I have everything I need to be a great mother.

I will seek help and
support when I need
it.

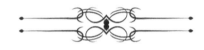

I am grateful for the
joys and wonders of
motherhood.

I am filled with hope and excitement for the future.

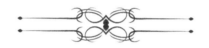

I am confident in my ability to provide a healthy environment for my baby.

I am surrounded by inspiration from other mothers.

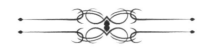

I trust my instincts and intuition to guide me in caring for my baby.

I listen to my baby's needs, and I respond with love.

I make choices that prioritize the health and well-being of my baby.

I am a good mother, and my child loves me.

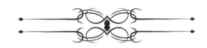

My baby knows all is well.

I was chosen to be the
mother of this child.

My baby is happy and
healthy.

My child is loved.

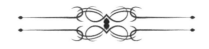

I am looking forward to the journey of motherhood that lies ahead.

THE POWER OF AFFIRMATIONS FOR LIFELONG WELL-BEING

Throughout this book, we've explored the incredible power of affirmations for supporting the physical, emotional, and spiritual well-being of both mother and baby during pregnancy and beyond. We've seen how positive self-talk can help you manage stress, build confidence, and deepen your connection with your baby.

By using affirmations regularly, you can create a foundation of love, positivity, and self-care that will serve you well throughout your life. Whether you're navigating the ups and downs of pregnancy and childbirth or facing new challenges in other areas of your life, affirmations can help you stay centered, grounded, and focused on your goals.

Remember that affirmations are not just words on a page—they are powerful tools that can transform your mindset. As you continue on your journey through motherhood and beyond, keep using affirmations to support your growth, nurture your relationships, and create a life that is filled with love, joy, and abundance.

Thank you for joining me on this journey, and I wish you all the best in your pursuit of lifelong well-being.

The Only Things Worth Having Are Not Things.

Dear Valued Customer,

We hope that you have found our book, "Daily Affirmations for Your Pregnancy & Childbirth", to be helpful and uplifting during your pregnancy journey. Our goal is to support and encourage expectant mothers and help them feel confident and empowered throughout their pregnancy.

If you have enjoyed the book and found it to be beneficial, we would greatly appreciate it if you could take a moment to leave a review on Amazon. Your feedback will help others discover the book and make informed purchasing decisions. It will also contribute to the continued success and growth of our work.

Thank you for your support and for taking the time to share your thoughts with us. We truly appreciate it!

Wishing you all the best in your pregnancy journey,

Serena A. Williams
Get Your Head Right Series

ABOUT THE AUTHOR

Serena A. Williams is an author and entrepreneur who was born in Brooklyn, NY. She currently resides in Maryland, where she has lived for over 20 years. Serena is a single mother of three adult children and has always been passionate about personal development and growth. Alongside her full-time job at a local university, Serena has spent the past decade studying and practicing affirmations as a means of improving her own life.

With a desire to share her knowledge and experience with others, she has authored the book "Affirmations for Your Pregnancy & Childbirth", providing a powerful resource for women seeking to cultivate self-love, self-care, and positive self-talk during pregnancy, childbirth, and beyond. Serena's dedication to personal growth and her passion for empowering others make her a valuable resource for anyone seeking to enhance their own life journey.

Made in United States
Troutdale, OR
12/26/2023